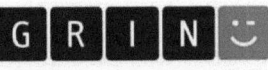

Healthcare Concepts for Women in India. Problems of the System and Ways to Solve Them

Navrup Kaur

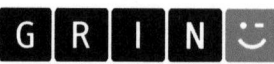

Bibliographic information published by the German National Library:

The German National Library lists this publication in the National Bibliography; detailed bibliographic data are available on the Internet at http://dnb.dnb.de.

ISBN: 9783346465245
This book is also available as an ebook.

© GRIN Publishing GmbH
Nymphenburger Straße 86
80636 München

Print and binding: Books on Demand GmbH, Norderstedt, Germany
Printed on acid-free paper from responsible sources.

The present work has been carefully prepared. Nevertheless, authors and publishers do not incur liability for the correctness of information, notes, links and advice as well as any printing errors.

GRIN web shop: https://www.grin.com/document/1041490

5. Semester Betriebswirtschaftslehre

Seminararbeit in:

Seminar Wirtschaft

über das Thema:

An overview of Health care concepts for women in India

Von

Kaur, Navrup

Abgabedatum: 15.01.2021

Table of Contents

Table of Figures

1. Introduction

"Over Two Lakh Young Girls Die Every Year in India Because of Their Gender"[1]. These are only figures concerning abortions and the death of girls under the age of 5. Far more women and girls die because of poor access to medical care or hygiene problems. Not to mention deaths due to domestic and sexual violence. Inequality is a very present issue in India. Not only is the woman disadvantaged in social and legal matters, but also in health aspects, the woman receives less attention for her concerns. Why is a lack of health care far more dangerous for women than it is for men?

This paper focusses on the issue of cultural misogyny and how this effects the health of women's' in India. It mainly analysis the structural and cultural problems, that directly affect the women's health. Therefore, the second chapter outlines the most important facts and figures of the sub-continent. In the third chapter the structure of the health system is discussed in further precision. The National Health Plan (NHP) is examined in more detail, and the structure and role of the healthcare centers is explained. The chapter ends with information about the National Rural Health Mission (NRHM) that was created to accompany the National Health Plan, which therefore focuses more intensively on the conditions of rural areas. In more bucolic regions and hard-to-reach places, the access to medicine is difficult. Women and girls in particular are dependent on male members of the family, as they are usually never educated or do not have the opportunity and permission to travel alone. These problems and many others that women have to endure are addressed in the following chapter. Women are immensely disadvantaged because of their gender. This relates both to the cultural aspect and the role of women and runs through the health sector. Hygiene, violence and pregnancy are dangerous factors for Indian women due to lack of education and the patriarchal society.
In this regard, both some state programs and private organizations have been trying to educate and support women in their position. For this purpose, numerous concepts have been developed to support women in the respective problem areas. Concepts, which go beyond the health-related, are to enlighten women and to help to overcome misogyny in this area retroactively and future-oriented.
The concepts are evaluated in the last chapter with regard to their effect, achievement of objectives and acceptance. It will be attempted to clarify whether the individual concepts are useful and to what extent they could perhaps even be improved.

This topic has a personal significance for every woman in the world and even more so for Indian women who have grown up in better circumstances outside India. Writing this paper is a way of understanding the contexts better it is about openly addressing the issue in the hope of being another voice demanding change in order to make India safer for women in every way. The following lines are an attempt to draw attention to terrible conditions and to change them. The paper is about thoroughly understanding the issue and lying out a base for further studies. Those may help implementing new local projects by combining the most effective aspects of the analyzed concepts.

---

[1] *Khullar. 23.05.2018*

2. The most important data about India

India is the seventh-largest country in the world in terms of area, but second in terms of population. The total area is 3.287.263 km², which is composed of 2.973.193 km² land area and 314.070 km² water surface.[2] The population in India is higher than ever before, with around 1.403 billion[3] people currently living on the subcontinent. Around 77,000 babies are born every day, but at the same time only 28,000 people die each one day. So the population is still growing. One big reason for this is the demographic change.
But it is growing into a certain direction, there are lot more man than women. The sex ratio of India is so alarming, that it is ranked 189th out of 201 countries.
There are 108,176 men for every 100 women. This makes a gender difference of 48.04% female to 51.96% male population.[4] This discrepancy derives from a strong cultural inequality and discrimination of women. Especially in rural areas, the gap is much bigger, the birth of a woman is considered negative in the culture of most Indians.
India's geography has 2,980,489 km² of rural land.[5] This accounts for nearly 90% of the total area. For this purpose, a rural area is defined by the Reserve Bank of India (RBI) as, an area with less than 49,000 inhabitants.[6] This means that around 66% of the people in India live in rural regions.[7] In most cases, they include villages that have the following characteristics: Most often, they have a population density of fewer than 400 people per km². The villages have clearly measured boundaries but usually have their small community council, also called "Panchayat". Most often, more than 75% of the men work in agriculture or other manual labor, such as pottery, tailoring, or sewing.
These small manual labor jobs and family businesses unfortunately do not bring much salary. India is one of the 40 poorest countries in the world. In terms of the number of people earning below the poverty line, India ranks first. About 270 million people live on less than $1.90 per day, and as many as 1.1 billion people live below $5.5 per day. That makes almost 80% of the total population.[8] The poverty line that is set, is barely enough for all three meals for one person, not to mention other essentials. This salary is of course far too low, especially for women, considering that they usually take care of children. So there is often no budget for any hygiene items that women would be needing.
Not only is there a lack of money, in Indian culture women struggle immensely and are oppressed in many ways. The topic of their health, for example, is not given much attention and evolves around many topics that are still considered taboo today. Women are seen inferior to men, which is a large human rights issue. In Western culture this inequality is less severe. Many topics that are taboo in India are addressed as early as school age, whereas sex education in India is hardly talked about.

---

[2] Cf. Länderdaten
[3] Cf. Department for Global and Social Contacts of Religious Nations, Status: 30.11.2020
[4] Cf. Ministry of Statistics and Programme Implementation & UN. 18.03.2020
[5] Cf. World Bank. Status: 2010
[6] Cf. Dhanlaxmi Bank Limited. 01.12.2010
[7] Cf. World Bank. Status: 2019
[8] Cf. Afus199620. 25.06.2020

3. Indian Health System

In the following section, the structure of the Indian health care system is roughly explained. The pronounced goal of the Indian government is to strengthen its health care system in the country and to provide access to medical facilities throughout India. For this purpose special concepts have been established to enable a more systematic development of the medical infrastructure. In the following the most important aspects of the National Health Plan and the National Rural Health Mission are discussed.

3.1 The General structure of the Indian healthcare system

Just like the German health care system, the Indian system is officially committed to the right to life and health. Health is considered a public good and is one of the basic human rights that should be accessible to everyone. The government's proclaimed goal is to provide basic health care to the people of India regardless of class, wealth, or location, and to make essential medical services available to everyone without financial hardship.

The organization of the health system is divided between the central government and the 29 federal states with the seven additional union territories. The federal states are independently responsible for the provision of health services. The state, on the other hand, regulates international contracts, medical education, food prevention, national disease control, and family planning programs.

The idea that health insurance should serve to cover the general population in the event of illness is such a huge task and by far not yet fulfilled. In 201 71.6% of expenditures in the health sector were financed by private funds. Therefore only 26.7% were due to the taxpaying population. However, the problem is that about 80% of the population lives below the poverty line, meaning they live on less than 6 U.S. dollars per day. In numbers, this means that only 36 million, or 27% of the people, are registered in a health insurance system at all. Private health insurance is also available, but only a small number of the urban, affluent population can afford and take advantage of it. Besides, there are some free programs for the entire population. These are intended to contain widespread diseases such as HIV, dengue fever, and malaria. Mothers and children are immunized against these and other common diseases. However, the availability of medical personnel, equipment, and medicines varies enormously within the different districts.

The only safety net for the population living in poverty is a series of government-funded centers that provide partial or total health care for some patients.

The government's current goals are to provide nationwide funding for medical supplies and to provide even greater security for health care in rural areas. Besides, there should be a reform of the health insurance system that entails a stronger social approach and prevents the already poor rural population from plunging into ever-higher costs just to be able to obtain basic health care. Some of the options introduced to provide universal health care are described in rudimentary form below.[9]

3.2 National Health Plan

To look at the issue as a whole and, one needs to look at how the healthcare system is set up there. To do this, we look at the infrastructure of the healthcare system and take a closer look at NHRM.

Health policy underwent a small revolution in 1964 when for the first time in India a real system emerged from the "Health Survey and Development Committee". In this committee, it was proposed to create a three-tier system, with prevention and cure playing an important

---

[9] Cf. Herter. 2018. P. 3

role in both urban and rural areas. It was planned to decrease the number of private doctors in favor of public ones, whereas the topic of health was supposed to be a lot more in political and social hands. This was to ensure that everyone received primary care regardless of individual socioeconomic conditions. The problem that arose, however, was that the capacities of public health care facilities were not sufficient and thus the gap was filled by private clinics. In 1983, a National Health Plan (NHP) was developed based on these goals. It was aimed that through referral systems and simple technologies, with the help of voluntary medical staff, everyone was supposed to be able to receive medical treatment by the year 2000. In 2003, a renewed form of the NHP was established to operate based on the NHP of 1983. This plan took advantage of the private sector and favored a decentralized form of decision-making, establishing more Western medicine.

Today, the health care system is multi-layered. The private sector has established itself primarily in urban areas and provides secondary and tertiary care. In rural areas, a three-tier system has been vested, which is adapted to the respective regional population norms. They are adjusted to the environment and cultural conditions.

Some centers that maintain the medical infrastructure in India have been established to provide primary health care to the smallest possible areas in India. These are listed and briefly explained below.[10]

3.2.1 Sub-Centers (SC)

Sub-Centers are set up where there is a population of only 5000 people or in mountainous areas of up to 3000 or areas that are difficult to reach. They provide a bridge to primary care, giving many a chance to survive until they reach a proper hospital where they can finally be treated. These centers offer the first possible contact with medicine for most people. The requirements for such a center are to have at least one male and one female health worker. Either the female health worker is already trained as a midwife or one must always be available at short notice. In the "Indian Public Health Standards (IPHS) Guidelines for Sub-Centers Revised 2012"[11] you can even find a complete list, from staff to equipment, of what is needed to set up such a center. "All "Minimum Assured Services" or Essential Services as envisaged in the Sub-center should be available, which include preventive, promotive, few curative and referral services [...]".[12]

3.2.2 Primary Health Centers (PHC)

The next level in the health system is the Primary Health Center. These are established for every 30,000 inhabitants or for 20,000 inhabitants in areas that are difficult to access. They must have a medical officer who can perform minor procedures and initiate both curative and diagnostic procedures. In addition, he*she takes the leading role in the primariy health center. Also, he*she takes the leading role in the primary health center. In addition to the doctor, there are usually up to 14 medical staff on site. There must be at least 5-6 beds for patient treatment and a place to stay for aftercare. The PHC is the link between the SB and the next level of healthcare.

3.2.3 Community Health Center (CHC)

Community health Centers are built at a population density of 120,000 inhabitants and in hard-to-reach areas for up to 80,000 inhabitants. Requirements for the staff are to have a team of 4 medical specialists on site. This includes a pediatrician, obstetrician or gynecologist, a physician, and a surgeon. Also, about 21 assistants have to be available as support. Facilities such as a delivery room, operating room, laboratories, and x-ray equipment must be at the CHC, along with an additional 30 beds for patient intake. Patients

---

[10] Cf. Chokshi et al. 07.12.2016. P. 9ff
[11] Cf. Azad et al. 2012
[12] Azad et al. 2012. P. 1

from PHC can be admitted, receive specialist consultations and obstetric care at this center. A significant positive increase can be seen in this regard. Since 2010, the number of CHCs under state management has increased from 91.6% to 99.3% in 2019, which were 5.335 centers in rural areas.[13]

3.2.4 First Referral Units (FRU)

A first referral unit has to provide a 24/7 emergency service in order to be considered an FRU. This includes first aid for newborns and other emergency cares. In addition, an FRU must be able to handle the usual hospital activities that come with an emergency. Three important points that such a unit must fulfill is to ensure emergency surgery for births, such as a cesarean section. In addition, the care and follow-up of newborns and thirdly, a blood reserve supply 24/7.[14] It must offer over 30 beds. Fresh drinking water and electricity must be available throughout, which is not a given everywhere in India. There must also be an ambulance facility. First referral units can usually provide adequate treatments to meet the needs of patients without being unnecessarily expensive.

In the following figure (refer to figure 1), the pyramid shows how the levels of the Indian healthcare system are structured. According to the number of centers and their equipment and size, the pyramid goes from the base of many but small sub-centers to the large but few district hospitals and medical colleges. In 2016, the number of facilities was 722 district hospitals, 4,833 CHCs, 24049 PHCs, and 148,366 SCs in India.[15] Lakhs is an Indian unit for 100,000.

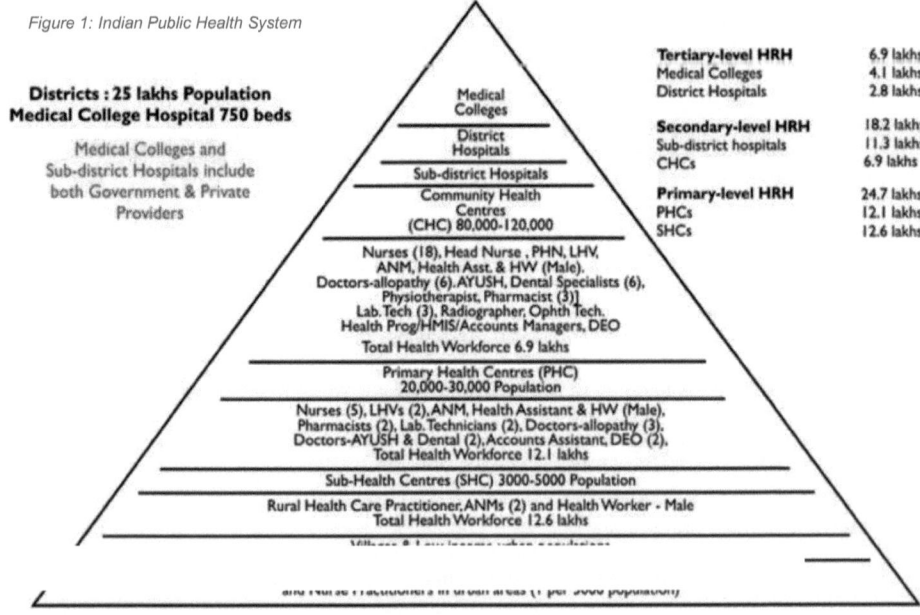

Figure 1: Indian Public Health System

Source 1: Health systems in India. Journal of Perinatology. 07.12.2016

https://www.ncbi.nlm.nih.gov/pmc/articles/PMC5144115/

---

[13] Cf. https://vikaspedia.in/health/health-directory/rural-health-care-system-in-india
[14] Ebd.
[15] Ebd.

3.3 National Rural Health Mission

To reduce neonatal mortality and birth complications for mothers and their children, the National Rural Health Plan was launched in 2005. It was targeted for 7 years, up to 2012. The achievement of the goals should be furthered by involving the communities, creating jobs, and making health accessible to everyone as quickly as possible. Hereby minimizing inequality through status, money, and gender. At the same time, this plan was intended to provide communities with access to drinking water, education, nutrition and also sanitation. Particular attention was paid to 18 states that tend to have weaker access to health care or lack adequate infrastructure, for example, due to poverty or inaccessibility. Public spending of the health system should be increased from 0.9% to 2-3% of GDP. In addition to hiring new medical staff under government salaries, not only new jobs should be created, but also new study places. Old centers were renovated and new ones built, so that medical sites were expanded and made accessible to more people. Smaller health committees in villages should be empowered to be accessible at the local level for health needs and to make decentralized decisions. In addition, patient advocacy committees at the village level are supposed to support health systems. IT systems support is supposed to enabled tracking of service delivery by and for mothers and children.

Thus, the NRHM had to fulfill the following tasks:
- Ease access to health facilities and utilization of quality health services.
- Create a collaboration between the central government, states, and local governments.
- Establish a forum for the involvement of Panchayati Raj Institutions and the community in the management of primary health programs and infrastructure.
- Promote equity and social justice.
- Establish a process that provides flexibility to states and the community to promote local initiatives.
- Develop a framework to promote intersectoral convergence for promotive and preventive health care.[16]

Therefore, about $17 billion US dollars were spent on this over a period from 2005 to 2013.[17] The government also plans to invest the equivalent of about 161 billion euros in rural development. The new health plan is intended to provide better health care for around half a million of India's poorest citizens. In the future, they will have up to 7,294 € per year at their disposal for hospital visits, promised Finance Minister Arun Jaitley in 2018.[18] Previously, the maximum was 377€. In 2018, 3.6% of GDP[19] was spent on healthcare in India. In 2019, it was as high as 3.89%. However, only 1% of this was actually invested from the government coffers, with the rest coming from private sources.[20]

In this table you can see the requirements that were to be fulfilled in the first 4 years by individual states and by the country itself. A proper schedule was drawn up, which the government felt was appropriate and achievable at the time.

Figure 2: Time Line for NRHM Activities

	Activity	Phasing and timeline
1.	Trained ASHA for every 1000 population	50% by 2007 - 100% by 08
2.	Health and Sanitation Comm. constituted in 600K villages & untied grants	30% by 2007 - 100% by 08
3.	2 Sub Health Centers strengthened/ established in 175K places	30% by 2007 - 60% by 09 - 100% by 10
4.	30K PHCs strengthened/ established with 3 Nurses	30% by 2007 - 60% by 09 - 100% by 10
5.	6.5K CHCs strengthened/ established with 7 Specialists and 9 Staff Nurses	30% by 2007 - 50% by 09 - 100% by 12
6.	1,8K Sub Hospitals strengthened to provide quality health services	30% by 2007 - 50% by 10 - 100% by 12

---

[16] Cf. Ministry of Health and Family Welfare. 2005
[17] Cf. Chokshi et al. 07.12.2016. P. 9ff
[18] Cf. Der Standard. 01.02.2018
[19] Cf. Radtke. 16.12.2019
[20] Cf. Wikipedia. 11.01.2021

7.	600 District Hospitals strengthened for quality health services	30% by 2007 - 60% by 09 - 100% by 12
8.	Hosp. Development Committees established in all CHCs, SDH, D. Hosp.	50% by 2007 - 100% by 09
9.	Prepared Health Action Plan for each district of the country	50% by 2007 - 100% by 08
10.	Untied grants for all villages medical Centers to promote health action	100% by 2008
11.	Annual maintenance grant for Centers, One Time support to RKSs at D. Hosp.	50% by 2007 - 100% by 08
12.	State and District Health Society established functional with requisite management skills	50% by 2007 - 100% by 08
13.	Systems of community monitoring put in place	50% by 2007 - 100% by 08
14.	Untied grants provided to each Village for Procurement and logistics to ensure availability of drugs and medicines at Sub-Centers/ PHCs/ CHCs	50% by 2007 - 100% by 08
15.	Centers & Hospitals fully equipped to develop intra health sector convergence coordination and service guarantees for family welfare & disease programs, etc.	30% by 2007 - 50% by 08 70% by 09 - 100% by 12
16.	District Health Plan reflects the convergence with wider determinants of health: e.g. drinking water, sanitation, women's empowerment, child development etc.	30% by 2007 - 60% by 08 100% by 09
17.	Facility and household surveys carried out in each and every district	50% by 2007 - 100% by 08
18.	Annual State and District specific Public Report published	30% by 2008 - 60% by 09 - 100% by 10
19.	Institution-wise assessment of performance against assured services	30% by 2008 - 60% by 09 - 100% by 10
20.	Mobile Medical Units provided to each district of the country.	30% by 2007 - 60% by 08 - 100% by 09

Source 2: Ministry of Health and Family Welfare
https://nhm.gov.in/WriteReadData/l892s/nrhm-framework-latest.pdf

To encourage state goals, the NRHM rewarded states for achieving goals. This was intended to encourage and empower individual states to invest even more time and money in their health care devices. Values from 2005 were compared to the actual states at that time in 2010. This resulted in a disadvantage for the states that had already made a good start at the beginning. Therefore, the states were subdivided in their initial values to start with comparable values in 2005. The subdivision took place as follows:

- High Focus States under NRHM, i.e., the eight former EAG states and two other states belonged to the first category (Bihar, UP, MP, Chhattisgarh, Orissa, Jharkhand, Uttarakhand, Rajasthan, J&K, Himachal Pradesh). This excludes the North-Eastern states.
- In the second category, the eight High Focus states in the North-Eastern region were evaluated.
- The non-High Focus states were awarded in the third category.

Scores were given on four quantifiable criteria and corresponded to importance.

- Macro health sector indicators
- Physical capacity and service delivery outcomes in rural service centers
- Results in improving human resources in the health system
- Governance outcomes

The idea behind this NRHM assessment and award was to promote health systems and drive individual states to link their rural areas more closely to their health system or strengthen it locally. This was to provide easier access to medical centers for more rural areas. In this way, the overall health system in the country should perform better.[21]

---

[21] Cf. Ministry of Health and Family Welfare. 30.10.2010

4. The role of women in India

Women make up 48% of the Indian population. Women take on the role of daughter, wife and many other positions in the family. Being a woman has a very different meaning in India than in some other Western countries. These differences are culturally very apparent and they subsequently have a strong impact on women's health. In the field of medicine gender differences disadvantage women in many ways. Some of the problems, both cultural and health wise, that women have to face are explained below.

4.1 Cultural role

Women are not considered equal to men in Indian culture. Even though already many improvements have been made in terms of equal rights, it is clear that centuries of cultural thinking cannot be easily removed from people's minds through enlightenment and modernization. The costs associated with a woman, whether born into the family or later as a married wife, makes her a burden in those kinds of societies, where women are economically strongly dependent. Even today, the Indian woman is raised to be a good wife and to play her role in the future household appropriately, i.e. she is supposed be able to do household chores and be obedient. Only in rare cases, time or money is invested into a girl, so that women often are neither educated, nor able to can pursue individual dreams and happiness.

In fact, with the birth, the dowry of the daughter is started to be accumulated, which is usually required for the wedding. In the past, this dowry served as a security reserve for herself, but since the British colonial period, it has been paid to the groom's family itself, increasing her economical dependencies. Until today thousands of women and girls are disowned, beaten, harassed, or even burned to death every year because of dowry disputes.[22] Even abortions in the womb result in India currently "missing" 63 million women.[23] The imbalance of men and women is huge and hard to decrease. For this reason, the practice of dowry has been prohibited by law in India since 1961. Despite this, 2 million girls are still killed each year.[24] The fact that women do not receive any education means that, in most cases, they are tied to the in-laws for the rest of their lives and are dependent on their husbands and society. Around 64.37% of Indian women aged 15+ are recorded as illiterate in 2018.

But even after birth, a being daughter is difficult and has loads of disadvantages today. Around 64.37% of Indian women aged 15+ years are recorded as illiterate in 2018. [25] Due to the fact that women do not receive any education, they are in most cases bound to the in-laws for the rest of their lives and dependent on the husband and society. If a family manages to marry off a girl despite her dowry, she usually becomes a helper in the house of her husband's family. She serves to perform marital duties and has the duty to perform tasks such as cooking and cleaning in the household. But even in wealthier families, where a housekeeper is usually hired, a woman is often not allowed to have her own professions, because she has to fulfill the role of a mother and wife in its entirety. A woman must surrender to this burden, however, because they are usually not educated differently or have hardly any other perspectives. A divorced woman is usually an outcast or seen as the source of discord herself. To escape these humiliations, the majority of the female population endures violence, rape, and degradation. Shockingly, in 2016, 46.6% of women still thought it was okay to be beaten by their husband, no matter what reason he may have.[26]

---

[22] Cf. Dominguez. 17.09.2013
[23] Cf. Booth. 30.01.2018
[24] Cf. SOS Kinderdörfer Weltweit. 27.02.2018
[25] Cf. World Bank. Status: 2018
[26] Cf. World Bank. Status: 2016l

In addition to domestic violence, abuse against women, in general, is very common. Every day almost 89 women are raped and these are only the reported cases. In 2018, 33,977 cases of rape victims were reported. Over 70% of the victims are under 18 years old and 90% of the victims know their rapist. In most of them, this is namely one of the family members, acquaintances, the husband, a family friend, or someone known to the parents.[27] The closer the (family) relationship to the perpetrator is, the more of a taboo it is.

Most of the time the victims never get justice. As you can see in the picture, more and more complaints are filed, but the number of cases that actually go to court is alarmingly low. Not only that women are victims of rape, but also afterward they have to suffer very bad consequences. Many victims are rejected, humiliated by society, or even disowned by their own families. Mostly the woman or the girl is not seen as a victim but is branded as responsible for the deed herself. The victim shaming is very severe in India. Questions about why and at what time she was out are raised. Accusations that she was certainly not wearing appropriate clothes or having goaded boys are yet harmless.

There are multiple reasons for the few reports like the humiliation of the woman, a lot of them are traumatized, unable to speak about what has happened to them, they often feel guilty themselves, suffer from unbearable shame and fear of society. They are often being blamed for what has happened to them and blame it on themselves, too. Women often try to repress or deny to themselves what has happened to them There is hardly any support that most victims receive. Also, reported cases, are mostly stamped by corruption and with self-infliction of the victim and swept under the carpet.

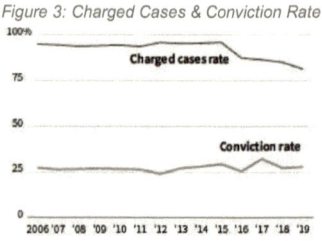

Figure 3: Charged Cases & Conviction Rate

Source 3: Reuters
https://www.reuters.com/article/us-india-rape-factbox-idUSKBN1YA0UV

India has a very misogynous culture. One term that sums up the male view of women is misogyny. While this is widespread throughout the world, it is very pronounced in India. Misogyny describes the pathological hatred of men towards women. This contempt for the female sex is considered the oldest tradition in Indian culture. The woman is seen as a man's property and can be treated accordingly.[28]

Therefore have women not only physical violence to fear, but can be simply married off as a good. Marriage among underage girls is widespread. The reasons for this are usually the poor conditions of the family. A daughter who is married off early does not have to be taken care of and is therefore no longer a financial burden. The money can be invested in the boy of the family, who is seen as the pension provision of the parents. But the consequences that a girl has to bear are usually not considered. Through a forced marriage, the girls lose any right to education and are often held like maids at a young age. Many soon become pregnant, even though they are not yet fully mature physically. This often leads to lifelong damage to their health.[29]

No education but also sexual education, child- and forced marriages, violence against women, and many other reasons lead to women and girls having to live with many health consequences. Most women, but also men, lack education in those and in healthcare. All these social and cultural differences between men and women lead to problems that women usually have to face alone.

---

[27] Cf. Sumeda. 10.01.2020
[28] Cf. Varma. 09.01.2018
[29] Cf. Kluve. Andheri Hilfe

4.2 Problems for women in the health sector

Poor health care makes India a dangerous place to live for women. In addition to the causes already mentioned above, such as (sexual) violence, religious traditions, and human trafficking, India's poor healthcare system was ranked fourth.

Every 100,000 births alone, 130 women die due to lack of medical care. The health system is growing in India, but it is not developing according to the progress of medicine.

A woman's health needs to be strengthened in several areas and supported by aid. The following are the most widespread problems a woman must face in the Indian health care system.

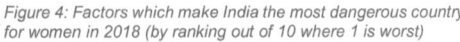
Figure 4: Factors which make India the most dangerous country for women in 2018 (by ranking out of 10 where 1 is worst)

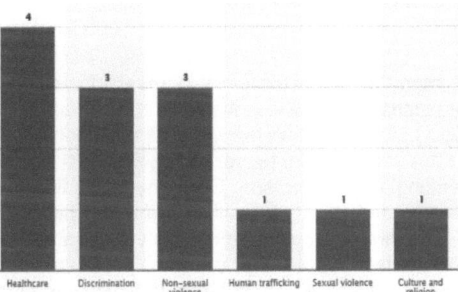

Source 4: Statista Research Department
https://www.statista.com/statistics/909596/india-most-dangerous-country-for-women/

4.2.1 A lack of menstrual hygiene

In their adolescence girls start menstruating which makes additional hygiene necessary. Most of the time, a girl does not receive proper education about what is happening to her body throughout her life. She has to face new experiences and changes herself. In most schools, sex education and topics concerning women and their bodies are not taught or not addressed at all. But since the majority of girls do not go to school, they don't even have a chance to be educated there. Even in the 21st century, gender issues are still taboo. They are popularly considered naughty and private, so most women never learn exactly how biology works in their bodies. They also never learn the proper way to deal with this issue at home. Because even there, mothers usually do not provide proper education.

71% of the girls have no knowledge about the topic before their own first period. Therefore, the girls struggle with a wide variety of feelings. A survey showed that 25% are in shock, 30% are scared, 70% are afraid and 22% even feel guilty and frustrated.[30]

Not only is the period considered a taboo subject, but in many cultures in India, a girl who has a period is regarded unclean. There are even villages where the girl has to leave her house during menstruation and live in a straw hut in the countryside for a few days. As a result, they are unprotected from men and very often even raped.

Besides not being educated, the girl must teach herself to keep herself hygienic. However, since most households lack the money to do so, women have to get creative to find an alternative for sanitary pads. In most cases, girls use old scraps of cloth, leaves, or shells that are used as protection. Often, however, these scraps cannot be cleaned thoroughly enough, so they are not hygienic. This results in infections, rashes, and discomfort. Nearly 70%[31] of girls and women in rural areas do not have access to sanitary products. A pack of sanitary napkins costs an average of 30-40 rupees[32], which most of the female population cannot even begin to afford every month.

Not only are domestic problems in terms of financing sanitary products more difficult, but access to toilets is not a given. In 2014, 40% of public schools could not boast separate

---

[30] *Cf. Geertz et al. 05.2016*
[31] *Cf. Chatterjee. 04.06.2020*
[32] *Cf. Garg et al. 20.04.2011*

toilets for boys and girls, and as many as 40% had no toilets at all.[33] As still, less than 50%[34] of the Indian population has access to clean water, and girls are forbidden to move freely during their period due to cultural rules, girls do not have many opportunities to clean themselves. Thus, a simple problem in the western region can lead to life-threatening diseases for girls and women in India.

4.2.2   A lack of maternal healthcare

In many places a too great number of mothers and children still die due to old-fashioned practices and views, poverty, and poor access to health care. In 2019, 34.3% of children died before their fifth live year, as a proportion of live births.[35] India made it to second place in this regard in 2019, recording 824,000 children dying before the age of five in a global ranking. By comparison, Germany had a figure of 3,000.[36]

"Maternal mortality is considered a key health indicator and the direct causes of maternal deaths are well known and largely preventable and treatable."[37]

Problematic issues that arise for pregnant women must be divided into two age groups. Child brides face very different difficulties in pregnancy than women who become pregnant later on.

Girls who get pregnant between the ages of 15-19 have bodies that are still maturing. In most cases, their bodies cannot yet handle pregnancy and so most pregnancies result in complications that lead to the death of the young girls. Since child pregnancies are forbidden, they usually never receive the medical support they need. Also, pregnancies of very young girls tend to occur in uneducated and rural areas where western medicine is not widely available. They are usually underweight and malnourished, as they grow up in poor conditions and because of the mysoginist culture. The co-investigator of the study, "Teen pregnancy still a major challenge in India, strongly linked to child stunting," S. Scott, noted that "the strongest links between adolescent pregnancy and child stunting were through the mother's education, her socio-economic status, and her weight."[38]

Compared to adolescent pregnancies, pregnant women of usual age, at least 20, face very different issues. Most of the problems they encounter are postpartum. Complications like severe bleeding, infections, gestational hypertension, complications during delivery and mostly illegal and unsafe abortions, are the most common reasons that lead to maternal deaths. About 2/3 of deaths are due to these reasons. Some of these factors can be treated quite easily and inexpensively. Bleeding, for example, is usually the result of severe iron deficiency, which can be easily treated with tablets.

Autonomy and self-determination correlate with the decision to seek care. Women who have enough decision-making power take the initiative and take care of prenatal and postnatal care, or receive the appropriate support. In many places, accessibility makes it difficult to reach medical facilities or to get there in time in labor. Women often do not have access to (public) transport or are not allowed to use it on their own and are therefore dependent on others. In many strictly religious households or where the woman lives in a large family, neither time nor financial resources are spent on them. Therefore, in a lot of areas, women give birth at home with a village midwife (Dai) and have no medical means available in case of complications.

---

[33] Cf. Geertz et al. 05.2016
[34] Cf. UNICEF: Program - Clean drinking water
[35] Cf. Urmersbach. 01.12.2020
[36] Ebd.
[37] UNICEF: Program – Maternal Health
[38] Sample. 15.05.2019

Besides the problems that directly affect the condition of women, there are also general problems that have an impact on their health. To begin with, India has the most privatized health care system in the world. This means that for individuals, medical services are much more expensive than most can afford. The cost of private treatment is so high that about 2-3% of the Indian population falls below the poverty line and therefore can't afford it. Government facilities are either inaccessible, poorly equipped, in poor condition, or overcrowded. 714 thousand beds were provided by the government sector in 2019. [39] Considering that 80% of India's population has to get by with 6 $ a day, it can be said that they can hardly use the private clinics. 80% of the population is 1.12 billion people, which means they are dependent on the government healthcare system. If you convert this, there are 1,570 people per hospital bed. In comparison, in Germany, there are only 125 inhabitants per bed. [40]

Not only are there not enough beds, but less than 25% of the Indian population has health insurance. I.e. they have to pay ad hoc for emergencies.
These reasons do not make it easy for the Indian society in general to use medical services, and even more so for a woman.
It is also to be considered that only 38% of the employees in the entire medical sector are female, in allopathic medicine even only 16%. Thus, because of cultural obligations, the woman does not have much choice. Either she is lucky enough to get a female assistant, or she is usually prohibited from medical assistance.

Furthermore, women also face many other (psychological) problems. India ranks 6th in the world in terms of the suicide rate among women. Nearly one in 15 women out of 100,000 population committed suicide in 2018. [41] Many of the reasons mentioned above, such as culture and victims of violence contributed to this high number.

Another big area that is very noticeable in India is the number of people with HIV. India has the third-largest HIV pandemic in the world. 2.1 million people had HIV in 2017, with 40% of those infected being women.[42] The reason for so many infected women is usually not them. In almost all cases, women got HIV from their husbands. Only in a few cases, the reason for infection was their own choice of several partners for private or professional reasons. And only in very rare cases, HIV is transmitted to the woman by uncleaned drug instruments. Thus, through cultural monogamy, it is usually never the woman who is to blame, but men who cheat on wives or women who are victims of sexual misconduct.
As a result, women have to struggle with the usual symptoms of HIV and AIDS but face much stronger stigmas. Affected women are usually disowned or isolated. Pregnant women are expelled from their families and can even infect their children. Therefore, there are other HIV support programs for women.

---

[39] *Cf. Statista. 2019*
[40] *Cf. Radtke. 13.08.2020*
[41] *Cf. WHO. Suicide Rate*
[42] *Cf. Avert. 28.01.2020*

5. Health Care Concepts

As India's figures on women, be it mother-child mortality rates, hygiene problems, or victims of violence, and sexual abuse perform very poorly in a global comparison, India increasingly became the focus of public attention. It was high time for Indian politics to bring a turnaround in the population. Since a revolutionary change in thinking is difficult to achieve, both the state and private institutions have to start providing support step by step. Over time these supports are supposed to, bring about a change in thinking and raise awareness about women and their health. In the following, different concepts of the private and state sector are illustrated, which should contribute to the support of female health. In This chapter exemplary concepts are analyzed.

5.1 Governmental health concepts for women

Women's health is no longer just a personal issue for each family, but is becoming an increasingly important factor in the economy of India. By strengthening women's health, the government aims to increase their participation in the economy. Some examples of government health programs are explained below.

Many of these concepts relate to first assistance for pregnant women and newborns. One of them is the Indira Gandhi Matritva Sahyog Yojana (IGMSY) conditional maternity benefit plan, which is a motherhood support scheme, was launched in 2010. It was introduced by the Ministry of Women and Child Development (WCD) and approved by the government as a pilot project in 52 districts. The project was about giving women a financial incentive if they sought medical support during and after pregnancy. The aim was to improve the nutritional and health status of women, especially during pregnancy and lactation, to create a better environment for them and their future children. In order to receive the 6,000 rupees grant, certain requirements had to be met by the women regarding pregnancy. By reducing the women's lost wages, long-term behavioral and attitudinal changes were to be induced.[43]
Similar to the previous concept, the Janani Suraksha Yojana (JSY) is also about mother-child care. It was introduced in 2012 with the National Rural Health Mission. The concept is to encourage rural women to give birth at medical centers in order to reduce maternal and neonatal mortality rates. Again, subsidies are distributed to women to encourage them to be more aware of their pregnancies and to minimize lost wages.[44]
Likewise, the Pradhan Mantri Surakshit Matritva Abhiyan (PMSMA) project assists in creating safe conditions for new mothers and newborns, in addition to providing support funds. The Pradhan Mantri Surakshit Matritva Abhiyan offers free tests such as blood pressure, sugar level, weight, hemoglobin tests, blood tests and screenings to pregnant women in the second trimester, in poorer areas.[45]

One project that is more supportive of adolescent girls is Sanitease. Founded by the Union Ministry of Youth Affairs and Sports in 2017, the project aimed to provide girls access to sanitary products. In schools, especially in rural areas, girls were given free sanitary pads monthly for their periods. It was first financed by support money from the government and subsequently by donations. [46] In addition, the Menstrual Hygiene Scheme (MHS) went beyond this. Here, in addition to the above-mentioned goals, the expansion of sanitary facilities and access to clean water were promoted. In collaboration with other projects, this

---

[43] Cf. Ministry Women and Child Development. 2010
[44] Cf. Ministry of Health and Family Welfare. 12.04.2005
[45] Cf. Manjunath. 14.11.2018
[46] Express News Service. 04.10.2017

project was introduced in 2011 and targeted girls in the 10-19 age group. The aim was to improve girls' hygiene and prevent health risks, as well as to raise awareness about menstruation.[47]

In 2011, a program: The Rajiv Gandhi Scheme for Empowerment of Adolescent Girls (RGSEAG) Sabla, was initiated by the Ministry of Women and Child Development. This program aimed to achieve the following aspects:
- the empowerment and self-development of adolescent girls
- to remedy malnutrition and strengthen their health
- Provide education in areas such as health, hygiene, nutrition, and sex education
- increasing household skills, life skills, and vocational skills
- educate girls in school and non-school subjects
- consultation of the possibilities of public services

This program was designed to support girls between the ages of 11 and 18 who, for various reasons, have not had the opportunity to go to school. Several institutions were involved in order to cover the different topics of this project and to pursue a common goal - the empowerment of Indian girls.[48]

5.2 Non-Governmental concepts for women

Because India is such a large and spread out country, with the second most inhabitants in the world, private organizations in addition to the government have made it their goal to improve health in India.

One of the most revolutionary innovations made Arunachalam Muruganantham. This man helped women in several areas through his invention. He invented a machine that enabled women to produce and resell self-manufactured sanitary napkins for their villages. He sold low-cost machines to underdeveloped rural areas, where he encouraged women to open small, independent factories. Muruganantham thus not only promoted women's health and hygiene by making sanitary napkins affordable at a fraction of the market cost, but he also empowered women financially. Women became more independent through his invention by being able to sell sanitary napkins themselves and earn their own wages. His invention led to the fact that women in the villages were more concerned with the taboo subject of menstruation and more awareness was awakened to this topic.[49]

WHO wanted to address a completely different target group with its plan. As mentioned above, violence against women is a major issue in India. But how they are treated afterward is often not less terrible than the offense itself. Medical helpers are often the first professional contact for survivors. At times, but still often enough today, the treatment of sexual victims has been condescending, insensitive, and degrading. Phrases such as "Another curse has landed. They do what they want, and then they come to us."[50], were not entirely uncommon. Almost always, victims lived in shame and were deemed self-responsible and never seen as victims. In order to make this interaction and first contact more comfortable for victims and to allow for a more sensitive approach, WHO issued a guide for healthcare providers to respond in 2011. In many cases, medical staff could do nothing but send the victims home after the appropriate examinations. The guide helped to train the staff to respond mentally to the women and perhaps to take further steps against the violence. In this way, the WHO

---

[47] Ministry of Health and Family Welfare. 2011
[48] Cf. Wikipedia. 02.12.2020
[49] Cf. Venema. 04.03.2014
[50] WHO. 25.11.2019

wants to achieve that more and more victims of violence take legal action against the violence of their perpetrators, thus deterring others and reducing this problem. [51]

UNICEF is also trying to do its part to improve women's health in India. The organization set up a program to reduce malnutrition among women, and thus placed greater emphasis on the Women's Nutrition program as part of their main program of India's nutrition. Malnutrition goes through a vicious cycle especially among women, because women who are underweight themselves also give birth to underweight babies. Or girls who become pregnant without having mature bodies of their own give birth to malnourished children. The deficiency that prevails in the mother, especially before pregnancy and in the first trimester, is usually passed on to the child and is thus born with a deficiency at birth. Babies struggling with malnutrition usually have to struggle with malnutrition for the rest of their lives, and so the vicious circle is created.

To break this vicious cycle, UNICEF set up a plan to implement nutrition interventions for women across the country. The 5 steps included in the plan for pregnant women were as follows:

1. Improving nutrition and increasing food quantities in households with pregnant women.
2. Preventing micronutrient deficiency and anemia.
→ This includes providing iron, vitamin A, calcium and folic acid supplements, malaria vaccinations, drug education during pregnancy and access to iodized salt.
3. Enabling easier access to basic nutrition and health services.
→ In this step, mothers and fetuses will be monitored more closely for weight, and more care will be provided, especially for high-risk pregnancies.
4. Universal access to sanitation and drinking water, and education on hygiene and menstruation.
5. Support for women in family planning.
→ Pregnancies that are too early, too fast, and too close together can more often lead to maternal deaths, miscarriages, or complications with birth or children. To prevent this, UNICEF offers empowerment courses to educate women and teach them to stand up for their rights. The aim is for them to take family planning into their own hands and make it more health-oriented.[52]

By and large, all organizations, whether private or public, have a common goal and that is to get women's health in India to a globally comparable level. In order to finance their organizations, the large organizations receive their funds from the state coffers and taxes, and partly also from donations. The private programs, are mainly financed by donations from all over the world.

5.3 Concept evaluation

After looking at all the concepts and their different themes related to women's health, a better evaluation of each scheme is possible. In the following, the evaluation of the schemes will be discussed. In doing so, an attempt will be made to examine the aspects of impact, achievement of objectives and acceptance in more detail.

Looking at the concepts of financial support for pregnant women and nursing mothers, the question arises as to what extent they make sense. While this does not force women to work, it is doubtful whether it will really bring about a long-term change in thinking in Indian society. In addition, the project assumed that the women have the ability to easily get to a medical center. So that means if the woman did not get the help or permission to get to a

---

[51] Cf. WHO. 25.11.2019
[52] Cf. UNICEF: Program – Women's Nutrition

medical center, she did not get any support from the government. Also, it must be remembered that the oppression of the woman, most of the time also means that she does not have access to money in the household. So who can say if the support money was really used to provide for the woman during her pregnancy. As surveys by IGMSY showed, both after and before pregnancy, about 50% used the money to buy more food for themselves and the family. 25% could not even use the money properly for themselves, but had to give it to the head of the family. Whether this really contributed to the goal of relieving the woman's burden is questionable. This was even stated in the final report of the program.[53] In the short term, the project makes sense because it probably helped many women for a brief period. In the long term, the government cannot spend inexhaustible donor money on such projects and the output is too small and short-sighted. In addition, not enough education was given on what the money was supposed to be used for in the first place, as evidenced by what the women and their families spent it on.

Comparatively, the JSY results were also similarly successful. Problematic was the payouts to health activists who were rewarded for helping pregnant women deliver at medical centers. They received a second lower reward if they provided postnatal checkups, but these were not worthwhile because of the effort involved. As a result, more than 80% of women, almost twice as many as before, gave birth with medical assistance. In contrast, only 2.5% received follow-up care. Therefore, the mortality rate fell only from 140 to 109 maternal deaths in 100,000 births.[54] Because of these sources of error, even the numbers show that the project was not thought through in its entirety and therefore had little success.

The PMSMA goes a little beyond this, offering women free tests to ensure a safe pregnancy. However, since the project is still ongoing and still fairly current, the non-existent numbers can be used to infer how effective this project has been.

The Sanitease program, on the other hand, not only includes the provision of hygiene products, but also uses schools, especially in rural areas, to educate girls about menstruation. In addition, government funds and donations were also used to build sanitary facilities for the girls to enable better and private hygiene. The problem that can be seen with this program is that only the girls who went to schools were addressed or given the opportunity to have hygiene products. While this is a good start, it is important to remember that it is the girls who will be even more disadvantaged because they did not receive the opportunity to go to school.

This is exactly the problem that the RGSEAG program addresses. It aims to empower women in several areas. Girls who do not have the opportunity to go to school should be encouraged and supported. Not only aspects such as hygiene and nutrition are addressed, but also their opportunity for further education, access to public facilities is explained and many other aspects that should support the girls on their future path.

Looking at the private programs, A. Muruganantham has managed to help women make their own hygiene products and made them accessible at low cost. Not only can they use them themselves, they can also resell them cheaply so that they can help others and gain economic independence through a fixed salary.

Such programs are an opportunity to empower women in a future-oriented way, because they manage to combine health concerns and financial independence. Thus, women are strengthened in their personality and health.

What the WHO is trying to do is clearly more important than the treatment itself. The WHO is trying to change the attitude of medical staff, in other words, the society itself. The aim of their guideline was to provide better primary health care for victims of violence. However, emphasis was placed on changing the attitude of the staff, i.e. how they approach the victims. Disrespect and insults are usually reactions that make it even more difficult for

---

[53] Ministry Women and Child Development. 04.2017
[54] Bhuyan. 16.09.2015

victims to recover, or to confront them at all. Therefore, it is important to make this confrontation, especially from professional contact, in such a way that victims feel well taken care of. If medical personnel start to avoid mysogenic reactions and deal better with women, they can in turn educate more people and encourage women. This could cause more women to confront violence and even report it.

UNICEF is also doing its part to improve the health of Indian women. The positive thing about the concept of this institution is that it not only pays attention to improving the health of women. It tries to break the vicious circle of malnutrition. For this purpose, not only food is provided, but a comprehensive 5-point plan has been established. This involves the family of pregnant women, educates, and provides access to nutritional supplements and healthy food. In addition, training is provided on how family planning can contribute to a healthy pregnancy.

A program must therefore be designed with the future in mind, in addition to the actual goal. For this it is important to educate the society and the family around the woman and to modernize their way of thinking. Girls must be given a comprehensive opportunity for education and professional prospects. In the school sector, the family must be obliged to send their children to school, where various aspects such as respect and hygiene are taught. In this way, a girl can realize and develop herself in the future.

6. <u>Conclusion</u>

In conclusion, all the concepts are trying to protect the health of girls. Many people are trying to bring about change in India through different concepts. However, the health of girls and women is not just about the opportunities available to them, but rather the mindset of the women and their society around them.

This work shows how multifaceted India is. When setting up such projects, many factors must be considered that carry more weight than in some other countries. It should not be forgotten that India combines several cultures and religions. It has many languages, a wide variety of infrastructures and environmental areas, and is one of the most populous countries in the world. This means that concepts that want to advance women in India must consider that they have to receive both: psychological as well as medical support. Safe births, school education, (menstruation-) hygiene, occupation, economic independence, security, equality, health and education must be offered and ensured to Indian women.

Of course, the problem with this is influencing the mindset is very complex and difficult. Cultural rooting takes decades and generations of impulses and methods in order to create a visible change in the larger masses. That is why the nutritional support or even hygiene training are just the first steps that are helping but they are not addressing the root cause of the problem, which is a very misogynous culture, that treats women terribly. In the longer term, however, not only women need to be trained, but the male factor contributes a much larger role in how a woman's health progresses. The men and their way of thinking about women have to improved, too. Despite the prevailing equality in the constitution, women are rarely considered equal to men. Woman are often being viewed and treated as objects rather than human beings. Still, one of the biggest problems is that the fault is always sought in the woman when she is harassed. The mentality, even of older women, is passed on to their children and especially sons. That is why gender training has a much more important role in improving healthcare for women. Until the mindset of the majority changes, the role of the woman never will be given the same value as the man. In conclusion a good initiative would rather be the combination of educational courses for men and women, and the addition of medical support. But the health support should definitely go beyond providing medical needs.
After all, what good does it do for a woman, who is a victim of violence or who is menstruating, if she receives medical care but is still is excluded or considered inferior by society?

Consequently, any healthcare concepts should also have the vision to eliminate the misogyny from culture of India. This is in fact the root of many problems that women have to face. Once this mindset and hatred is shrunk, a woman can start basically from birth with the same (healthcare) conditions as a man.
It will be difficult to bring about this change in rural areas. Cut off from civilization, usually living only in their small community, a modern an open growth mindset is difficult to achieve. Therefore, among other aspects, the possibility of school education must be strongly emphasized. To this end, the government must implement a compulsory school system also for girls and boys and provide both financial and infrastructural opportunities for children to attend school. In this way, not only could education take place through biology classes, but equality and respect for women could be taught at a young age.

All these opportunities and rights are self-evident for the Western culture,but cannot be brought forth in one piece in Second World countries. Therefore, the right combination of government and private programs is important to achieve a common goal sooner. The future should be that no girl should have to fear banal things like having her period, being unworthy, or just being a girl. She should have the same rights as a boy, a right to education, a profession, or to be able to shape the future according to her will. Medical requirements should no longer be an obstacle for her. This paper is an invitation to dig deeper into better understanding and finding solutions for the problems that have been addressed through out.

7. References

Afus199620	Afus199620: Liste der Länder nach Armutsquote. Wikipedia. 25.06.2020. available at: https://xtools.wmflabs.org/articleinfo-authorship/de.wikipedia.org/Liste_der_L%C3%A4nder_nach_Armutsquote?us elang=de, last checked on: 15.01.2021
Avert	Avert: HIV and AIDS in India. 28.01.2020. available at: https://www.avert.org/professionals/hiv-around-world/asia-pacific/india#:~:text=In%202017%2C%2079%25%20of%20people%20living%20with%20HIV%20in%20India,child%20transmission%20(PMTCT)%20services, last checked on: 15.01.2021
Azad	Azad, Ghulam Nabi et al.: Indian Public Health Standards (IPHS) Guidelines for Sub-Centres. Directorate General of Health Services, Ministry of Health & Family Welfare. Government of India. 2012. available at: https://nhm.gov.in/images/pdf/guidelines/iphs/iphs-revised-guidlines-2012/sub-centers.pdf, last checked on: 15.01.2021
Bhuyan	Bhuyan, Ragini: The limited success of Janani Suraksha Yojana. Mint. 16.09.2015. available at: https://www.livemint.com/Opinion/PwRuPTCR8imbCM1mKbEJLK/The-limited-success-of-Janani-Suraksha-Yojana.html, last checked on: 15.01.2021
Booth	Booth, Samantha: Indiens fehlende Frauen. Märkische Allgemeine. 30.01.2018. available at: https://www.maz-online.de/Nachrichten/Wissen/Indiens-fehlende-Frauen, last checked on: 15.01.2021
Chatterjee	Chatterjee, Patralekha: Improving menstrual hygiene among adolescent girls in India. 04.06.2020. The Lancet. available at: https://ciniitalia.org/wp-content/uploads/2020/06/the-lancet-vol-4-issue-6-june-2020-article-CINI-menstrual-hygiene-among-girls.pdf, last checked on: 15.01.2021
Chokshi	Chokshi, M./ Patil, B./ Khanna, R./ Neogi, SB./ Sharma, J./ Paul, VK./ Zodpey, S.: Health systems in India. Journal of Perinatology. 07.12.2016. available at: https://www.ncbi.nlm.nih.gov/pmc/articles/PMC5144115/pdf/jp2016184a.pdf, last checked on: 15.01.2021
Department for Global and Social Contacts of Religious Nations	Department for Global and Social Contacts of Religious Nations: Indien Bevölkerungsuhr. Countrymeters. available at: https://countrymeters.info/de/India, last checked on: 15.01.2021
Der Standard	Der Standard: Indiens Regierung kündigt großzügige Ausgaben für Arme an. 01.02.2018. available at: https://www.derstandard.de/story/2000073443776/indiens-regierung-kuendigt-grosszuegige-ausgaben-fuer-arme-an, last checked on: 15.01.2021
Dhanlaxmi Bank Limited	Dhanlaxmi Bank Limited: Rural India: Where is It?. In focus. 01.12.2010. available at: https://www.dhanbank.com/pdf/reports/InFocus-December%201,%202010.pdf, last checked on: 15.01.2021
Directorate General of Health Services Ministry of Health & Family Welfare	Directorate General of Health Services, Ministry of Health & Family Welfare : Indian Public Health Standards (IPHS) - Guidelines for Sub-Centres Revised 2012 . 2012 available at: https://nhm.gov.in/images/pdf/guidelines/iphs/iphs-revised-guidlines-2012/sub-centers.pdf, last checked on: 15.01.2021

Dominguez	Dominguez, Gabriel: Mitgift in Indien: Eher Fluch als Segen. DW Akademie. 17.09.2013. available at: https://www.dw.com/de/mitgift-in-indien-eher-fluch-als-segen/a-17093170#:~:text=In%20Indien%20ist%20die%20uralte,im%20Zusammenhang%20mit%20Mitgift%2DStreitigkeiten, last checked on: 15.01.2021
Expat News	Expat News: Gesundheitssystem von Indien: Medizinische Versorgung in privater Hand. 03.11.2016. available at: https://www.expat-news.com/life-style/indien-medizinische-versorgung-in-privater-hand-28230#:~:text=Nur%2061%20Dollar%20pro%20Jahr%20f%C3%BCr%20die%20Gesundheit%20des%20Einzelnen&text=Tats%C3%A4chlich%20hat%20Indien%20das%20am,staatliche%20und%20private%20Gesundheitsausgaben%, last checked on: 15.01.2021
Express News Service	Express News Service: Women's health scheme 'Sanitease' launched. The Indian Express. 04.10.2017. available at: https://indianexpress.com/article/india/womens-health-scheme-sanitease-launched-4873312/, last checked on: 15.01.2021
Garg	Garg, Rajesh/ Goyal, Shobha/ Gupta, Sanjeev: India Moves Towards Menstrual Hygiene: Subsidized Sanitary Napkins for Rural Adolescent Girls—Issues and Challenges. Springer Link. 20.04.2011. available at: https://link.springer.com/article/10.1007%2Fs10995-011-0798-5, last checked on: 15.01.2021
Geertz	Geertz, Alexandra/ Iyer, Lakshmi/ Kasen, Perri/ Mazzola, Francesca/ Peterson, Kyle: Menstrual Health in India – Country Landscape Analysis. FSG. 05.2016. available at: https://menstrualhygieneday.org/wp-content/uploads/2016/04/FSG-Menstrual-Health-Landscape_India.pdf, last checked on: 15.01.2021
Herter	Herter, Anna-Lena: Vergleich des indischen und des deutschen Gesundheitssystems. Ayurvedische Medizin und Physiotherapie. GRIN. 2010. available at: https://www.grin.com/document/452741, last checked on: 15.01.2021
Khullar	Khullar, Amanat: Over Two Lakh Young Girls Die Every Year in India Because of Their Gender. The Wire. 23.05.2018. available at: https://thewire.in/women/gender-bias-under-five-mortality, last checked on: 15.01.2021
Kluve	Kluve, Heike: Zwangsheirat (Kinderheirat) gefährdet Zukunft von Mädchen. Andheri Hilfe. available at: https://www.andheri-hilfe.de/informieren/selbststaendigkeit-sichern/kinder-vor-kinderheirat-schuetzen/#:~:text=Zwangsheirat%20(Kinderheirat)%20gef%C3%A4hrdet%20Zukunft%20von,sind%20Gewalt%20und%20Unterdr%C3%BCckung%20ausgesetzt.&text=Damit%20z%C3%A4hlt%20Indien%20weltweit%20zu,Kinderheiraten%20-%20trotz%20des%20gesetzlichen%20Verbotes, last checked on: 15.01.2021
Länderdaten	Länderdaten: Flächendaten aller Staaten der Erde. 20.01.2013. available at: https://www.laenderdaten.de/geographie/flaeche_staaten.aspx, last checked on: 15.01.2021
Manjunath	Manjunath, Usha: 4 Healthcare schemes by the Government every woman must know. MyStory. 14.11.2018. available at: https://yourstory.com/mystory/4-healthcare-schemes-by-the-government-every-woman-fl6i4eq2ms, last checked on: 15.01.2021
Mentschel	Mentschel, Stefan & Sharma, C. Dinesh: Zwischen Versorgungsnotstand und Medizintourismus. BpB. 28.04.2014. available at: https://www.bpb.de/internationales/asien/indien/189184/indiens-gesundheitssystem, last checked on: 15.01.2021

Ministry of Health and Family Welfare	Ministry of Health and Family Welfare: National Rural Health Mission – Criteria For State Awards. 30.10.2010. available at: https://nhm.gov.in/WriteReadData/l892s/601511241464073617.pdf, last checked on: 15.01.2021
Ministry of Health and Family Welfare	Ministry of Health and Family Welfare: National Rural Health Mission. 2005. available at: https://nhm.gov.in/WriteReadData/l892s/nrhm-framework-latest.pdf, last checked on: 15.01.2021
Ministry of Health and Family Welfare	Ministry of Health and Family Welfare: Janani Suraksha Yojana. National Health Mission. 12.04.2005. available at: https://nhm.gov.in/index1.php?lang=1&level=3&sublinkid=841&lid=309, last checked on: 15.01.2021
Ministry of Health and Family Welfare	Ministry of Health and Family Welfare: Menstrual Hygiene Scheme (MHS). National Health Mission. 2011. available at: https://nhm.gov.in/index1.php?lang=1&level=3&sublinkid=841&lid=309, last checked on: 15.01.2021
Ministry of Statistics and Programme Implementation & UN	Ministry of Statistics and Programme Implementation & UN: Sex ratio of India. Statistics of Times. 18.03.2020. available at: http://statisticstimes.com/demographics/country/india-sex-ratio.php#:~:text=Sex%20Ratio%20of%20India%20is,males%20population%20than%20females%20population, last checked on: 15.01.2021
Ministry Women and Child Development	Ministry Women and Child Development: Indira Gandhi Matritva Sahyog Yojana (IGMSY) - a Conditional Maternity Benefit (CMB) Scheme. Social protection. 2010. available at: https://socialprotection.org/es/discover/publications/indira-gandhi-matritva-sahyog-yojana-igmsy-conditional-maternity-benefit-cmb, last checked on: 15.01.2021
Ministry Women and Child Development	Ministry Women and Child Development: Quick Evaluation Study on Indira Gandhi Matritva Sahyog Yojana (IGMSY). 04.2017. available at: http://niti.gov.in/writereaddata/files/document_publication/IGMSY_FinalReport.pdf, last checked on: 15.01.2021
Radtke	Radtke, Rainer: Anteil der Gesundheitsausgaben am Bruttoinlandsprodukt ausgewählter Länder 2018. Statista. 16.12.2019. available at: https://de.statista.com/statistik/daten/studie/283361/umfrage/anteil-der-gesundheitsausgaben-am-bruttoinlandsprodukt-ausgewaehlter-laender/, last checked on: 15.01.2021
Radtke	Radtke, Rainer: Krankenhausbetten in Deutschland bis 2018. Statista. 13.08.2020. available at: https://de.statista.com/statistik/daten/studie/157049/umfrage/anzahl-krankenhausbetten-in-deutschland-seit-1998/, last checked on: 15.01.2021
Reuters	Reuters Staff: Statistics on rape in India and some well-known cases. Reuters. 06.12.2019. available at: https://www.reuters.com/article/us-india-rape-factbox-idUSKBN1YA0UV, last checked on: 15.01.2021
Sample	Sample, Drew: NEW STUDY: Teen pregnancy still a major challenge in India, strongly linked to child stunting. IFPRI. 15.05.2019. available at: https://www.ifpri.org/news-release/new-study-teen-pregnancy-still-major-challenge-india-strongly-linked-child-stunting, last checked on: 15.01.2021
SOS Kinderdörfer Weltweit	SOS Kinderdörfer Weltweit: Mädchen in Indien weiterhin in Gefahr. 27.02.2018 available at: https://www.sos-kinderdoerfer.de/informieren/aktuelles/news/indien-maedchen-in-gefahr, last checked on: 15.01.2021
Statista Research Department	Statista Research Department: Factors which make India the most dangerous country for women in 2018 - (by ranking out of 10 where 1 is worst). Statista.

	16.10.2020. available at: https://www.statista.com/statistics/909596/india-most-dangerous-country-for-women/, last checked on: 15.01.2021
Statista Research Department	Statista Research Department: Estimated number of public and private hospital beds across India as of 2019. Statista. 16.10.2020. available at: https://www.statista.com/statistics/1128673/india-number-of-public-and-private-hospital-beds-estimated/, last checked on: 15.01.2021
Sumeda	Sumeda: Rapes in India: 94% offenders known to victim, every 4th victim a minor. India Today. 10.01.2020. available at: https://www.indiatoday.in/india/story/rapes-in-india-offenders-victim-minor-data-ncrb-1635691-2020-01-10, last checked on: 15.01.2021
UNICEF	UNICEF: Clean drinking water - Ensuring survival and improved outcomes across all outcomes for every child. available at: https://www.unicef.org/india/what-we-do/clean-drinking-water#:~:text=Less%20than%2050%20per%20cent,to%20safely%20managed%20drinking%20water.&text=Groundwater%20from%20over%2030%20million,water%20requirements%20in%20urban%20areas, last checked on: 15.01.2021
UNICEF	UNICEF: Maternal health - UNICEF's concerted action to increase access to quality maternal health services. available at: https://www.unicef.org/india/what-we-do/maternal-health, last checked on: 15.01.2021
UNICEF	UNICEF: Women's Nutrition. available at: https://www.unicef.org/india/what-we-do/womens-nutrition, last checked on: 15.01.2021
Urmersbach	Urmersbach, Bruno: Kindersterblichkeit in Indien bis 2019. Statista. 01.12.2020. available at: https://de.statista.com/statistik/daten/studie/753066/umfrage/kindersterblichkeit-in-indien/#:~:text=Im%20Jahr%202019%20betrug%20die,somit%20rund%203%2C04%20Prozent , last checked on: 15.01.2021
Varma	Varma, Amit: Misogyny is the oldest Indian tradition. BL Ink. 09.01.2018. available at: https://www.thehindubusinessline.com/blink/talk/misogyny-is-the-oldest-indian-tradition/article9800756.ece#, last checked on: 15.01.2021
Venema	Vinema, Vibeke: The Indian sanitary pad revolutionary. BBC World Service. 04.03.2014. available at: https://www.bbc.com/news/magazine-26260978, last checked on: 15.01.2021
Vikaspedia	https://vikaspedia.in/health/health-directory/rural-health-care-system-in-india
WHO	WHO: Suicide rate estimates, crude - Estimates by WHO region. available at: https://apps.who.int/gho/data/node.main.MHSUICIDE?lang=en, last checked on: 15.01.2021
WHO	WHO: Indian health workers transform care for women survivors of violence. 25.11.2019. available at: https://www.who.int/news-room/feature-stories/detail/indian-health-workers-transform-care-for-women-survivors-of-violence, last checked on: 15.01.2021
Wikipedia	Wikipedia: Healthcare in India. 11.01.2021. available at: https://en.wikipedia.org/wiki/Healthcare_in_India, last checked on: 15.01.2021
Wikipedia	Wikipedia: Sabla (India). 02.12.2020. available at: https://en.wikipedia.org/wiki/Sabla_(India)#:~:text=The%20Rajiv%20Gandhi%20Scheme%20for,of%20Women%20and%20Child%20Development, last checked on: 15.01.2021
Wikipedia	Wikipedia: Rural area. 14. 01 2021. available at: https://en.wikipedia.org/wiki/Rural_area#cite_note-dhanbank.com-15, last checked on: 15.01.2021

Wikipedia	Wikipedia: Women's health in India. 31.12.2020. available at: https://en.wikipedia.org/wiki/Women%27s_health_in_India, last checked on: 15.01.2021
World Bank	World Bank: India - Rural Land Area (sq. Km). Trading Economics. available at: https://tradingeconomics.com/india/rural-land-area-sq-km-wb-data.html, last checked on: 15.01.2021
World Bank	World Bank: India - Rural Population. Trading Economics. available at: https://tradingeconomics.com/india/rural-population-wb-data.html, last checked on: 15.01.2021
World Bank	World Bank: India - Adult Illiterate Population, 15+ Years, % Female. Trading Economics. available at: https://tradingeconomics.com/india/adult-illiterate-population-15-years-percent-female-wb-data.html, last checked on: 15.01.2021
World Bank	World Bank: India - Women Who Believe A Husband Is Justified In Beating His Wife (any Of Five Reasons). Trading Economics. available at: https://tradingeconomics.com/india/women-who-believe-a-husband-is-justified-in-beating-his-wife-any-of-five-reasons-percent-wb-data.html, last checked on: 15.01.2021

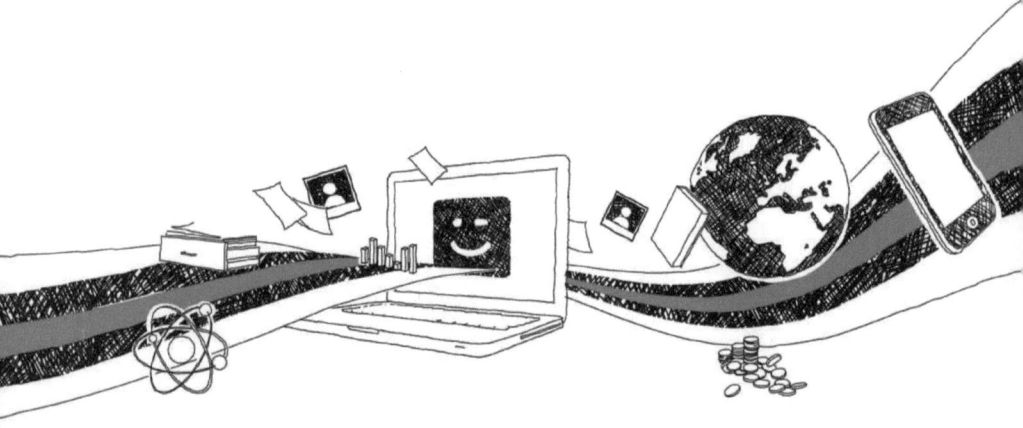
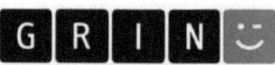